"Angels in the Valley"

By Patti SassyAngel Chiappa

This book is dedicated to all the angels who have a heart full of faith even though there going through their own valley. For all the wonderful care givers who encourage, love and give. For my dear friends and loved ones who have lost their battle to cancer. My great aunt Viola, uncle Walter, uncle Willie, uncle Al, uncle Joe, Diana, Kyle, Sherry, grandpa Fred and my beloved father Bernie, aunt Dot, great grandma, aunt Roberta, you are my angels in heaven. For aunt Dot and Jane who are still fighting there courageous battle. Your courage, strength, and light will always be a part of me. Thank you for being a true inspiration. For my loved ones who encouraged me about the idea for this book. Thank you for your support, patience, and listening ears. This book is for all of you. May these scriptures, poems, and prayers, bring you peace and comfort. A portion of the profits of this book will be donated to the Dana Farber Fund.

Chapter One

"But your dead, will live. Their bodies will rise. You who dwell in the dust wake up and shout for joy. Your dew is like the dew of morning. The earth will give birth to her dead. " Isaiah 26:19

The first time I heard the word cancer I was four years old. I did not know what the word meant but I knew there was a lot of pain associated with it. It was my fourth birthday. My family had gathered around my birthday cake. I remember as I blew out the candles my great aunt with her gentle blue eyes and soft smile began to cry. "I have breast cancer." She said.

I remember clearly looking around the room at my family member's faces that were just full of joy now looking lost, angry, and full of disbelief.

I remember turning to my great aunt. A woman that was so spiritual, so beautiful, so gentle, that I actually thought she was an angel and saying " What is cancer? "My great aunt the woman who taught me about prayer, faith, and forgiveness, took me by my little hand and tearfully said, "Cancer is a way God brings us closer to him. It is a way that God teaches us to rely on our faith. It is a way that God shows us how strong we really are. Cancer, darling is an illness that makes people sick but it also makes them cherish every moment, every sunrise, every sunset, every song they hear, every smile they see, every hug they give and receive, every kiss, every day."

I looked at my aunt and asked, "Are you going to die? "My aunt responded, "I may leave this earth but when I do, I don't want you to be sad because when I leave earth I will be starting my new life with Jesus in heaven."

"When Jesus entered the rulers house and saw the flute players and the noisy crowd he said,"Go away the girl is not dead but asleep, but they laughed at him. After the crowd had been put outside he went in and took the girl by the hand and she got up. " Matthew 9 :23 to 9: 25

After my fourth birthday my great aunt ended up in the hospital. She began receiving chemo treatment. She had lost weight, her hair, and her energy, but not her beautiful spirit. I remember clearly how whenever I saw her she would make me laugh. Her body had changed, but not her beautiful smile, her loving personality, and her gentle heart. I saw how my family had overcome the beast called cancer through faith, prayer and togetherness. Even at an early age I began to understand that cancer can never rob memories, a person's spirit, the love of family and friends, but most of all a person's faith. I understood that Jesus would stand by a person through good and bad, rain or sunshine, fear or faith.

The most important lesson I learned from my aunt was the same God on the mountain was the same God in the valley. I saw God through my aunt's eyes. I saw at her most desperate time of need that when she was reaching out to God, that he was reaching right back. "God will never leave you.", she said to me the last time I ever saw her. "No matter what happens God will never leave you. '

The night before my aunt died I had a beautiful dream. I was engulfed by peace and comfort when I saw my beautiful aunt healthy and happy walking arm and arm with Jesus. My aunt was wearing a long, flowing, white dress. Her hair was full and thick and in little curls. My aunt smiled at me saying, "By his stripes I am healed'. She then kissed me on the head.

I said, "Bye auntie."The next night my grandma and my godfather watched my great aunt take her last breath.

The day we buried my great aunt it was a beautiful spring day. New buds bloomed on trees, perfume from lilacs and roses peppered the air, and a bright yellow sun warmed our faces. I was seven. For three years my family had been ironically bonded even stronger by cancer. We had learned to make every day count, how to sacrifice, but most importantly how important it was to pray as a family.

It was April 23, 1981 and we said our final goodbyes to a woman who inspired us to life every day to its fullest. It was my aunt's battle with cancer that taught me the meaning of this scripture. From Luke 12 :8"I tell you who ever acknowledges me before man the son of man will also a acknowledge him before the angels of God."April 23, 1981, I did not weep for my aunt for I knew that she had left this earth but had started her new life with Jesus. My aunt Viola had never given up on prayer, never became bitter, or angry, or blamed God for her illness. She actually thanked God for allowing her to learn that cancer taught her how to be strong, and enjoy every moment of life with your loved ones.

Chapter Two

"Whatever happens abide steadfast in determination to simply cling to God.' St. Francis De Sales.

My grandfather Frederick was my hero. As a young man he worked selling pretzels in Madison Square Garden for just pennies a day. He was a stern German with a fighting spirit. He was a care giver, a male nurse during world war two. A husband that would sacrifice anything for his wife. A father who was devoted. A grandfather full of wonderful advice, a friend to all. He was also the second person close to me that was stricken with cancer.

My grandfather Fred was diagnosed with stomach cancer in the late 1980s. When he was diagnosed we just would not accept it. My grandfather was the patriarch of our family. He was a strong, brave man who was bigger than life with his hearty laugh, and booming voice. He was a warrior.

It was because my grandfather, was this strong manly man that our family just could not accept that cancer had claimed his cells. We together as a family declared war on my grandfather's cancer.

We changed my grandfather's diet, tried all the alternative medicines, prayed, and gave my grandfather's cancer over to God. We just would not let cancer claim him. Grandpa was just as determined to stay with us as we were determined of keeping him here. He was too stubborn to let cancer take him away from his family. Grandpa spent his days hiding his pain from us, so we would not fear.

We spent our days giving grandpa a reason to stay here.

"Strength is born in the deep silence of long suffering hearts, not amidst joy.' Felicia Hemans.

It was just before thanksgiving when my grandfather had part of his colon removed. The doctors had warned us that he may not survive the operation. But we laughed in the face of their warning. They did not know how big our God was or how strong my grandfather was. The day came for my grandfather's surgery. The whole family and our pastor gathered at the hospital. We spent seven hours praying while my grandfather went under the knife.

Almost eight hours passed when a tired and weary surgeon walked out of the or with tears in his eyes saying, "He made it, he made it.", in a joyful voice.

When we saw my grandfather in the recovery room in a horse and groggy voice he said, "I'm hungry".

We knew at that moment grandpa was going to be ok.

Our family celebrated Thanksgiving that year at a Long Island hospital. We ate Thanksgiving dinner off of plastic hospital trays, but it was our best Thanksgiving ever. My grandfather returned home only three days after having major surgery amazing all of his doctors.

It was one doctor in particular that was deeply touched by my grandfather's victory. A Jewish man, he had rejected the idea that Jesus existed all his life until he met my grandpa. So moved by the miracle he had saw, this doctor questioned my grandfather about his flawless faith. My grandfather had simply explained to him that is was easy to know Jesus existed because he saw him everywhere he looked. In the eyes of his loved ones, in the rain, in a flower, in the moon light. My grandfather had shared with this doctor his favorite scripture. " Those who know your name will trust in you for you Lord have never forsaken those who seek you." Psalm 9:10.

So astonished by my grandfather's healing this devoted Jewish man gave his heart to Jesus in the presence of a man who Jesus healed that had been stricken with stage three colon cancer. Later on this man brought his family to Christ also. My grandfather went on to have many happy and joyful years with our family. Grandma and grandpa got to celebrate their 50 anniversary renewing their vows in a beautiful , romantic ceremony. I will never forget it for as long as I live. It was Feb. 4, 1991, it was a snowy afternoon. My immediate family went to 5 o'clock mass with my grandparents. At a church my grandparents had attended for 40 years. My grandfather was an usher there and had arranged the whole ceremony without any of us knowing it. He had told mom, dad, my brother, and I to get dressed up because we were going out to dinner at our favorite restaurant Friendly's after church.

 My brother and I were very excited because we loved the ice cream there. We met my grandparents at church on that snowy afternoon. During the mass I noticed my grandfather was smiling from ear to ear.

After mass my grandfather sprang the surprise on all of us. The man who had survived brutal colon cancer got down on one knee and proposed to grandma all over again.

My grandma who was a little fireball standing at only five feet and weighing only 100 lbs. tearfully accepted, but then hit my grandfather playfully on his backside for not telling her what he was up too.

I got to be my grandmas maid of honor, and my grandfather had my brother as best man as we tearfully, joyfully, witnessed how a Christ centered marriage could endure the most testing trials, most pouring rains and most shaky roads.

My hears still swells with happiness as I recall how my grandfather called grandma his Florence Nightingale as he recited his wedding vows again. How after the beautiful ceremony was over he proudly told everyone present at the church how God truly healed him.

 For years after my grandfather won his battle with cancer, he got to enjoy building wonderful memories, he got to see his grandchildren graduate high school, dance many polkas with grandma and play many songs on his organ.

"Faith never knows where it is needed but it loves and knows the one who is leading."Oswald Chambers.

The second time my grandfather was diagnosed with cancer this time kidney we once again declared war.

This time my grandfather was much older and fragile then the last. None of us however believed that God would simply decide that it was time for grandpa to come home.

 My grandfather's health declined very quickly. It was a matter of weeks before he was bed ridden and my grandmother became a full time care taker. We all dealt with my grandfather's second battle with cancer in our own personal way. My grandmother was simply in denial, and sincerely believed that grandpa would get better. My dad ,my grandpa's only child took my grandfather's role as family patriarch very seriously and put on a brave face.

Some of us felt betrayed by God and became angry and hardened.

Personally I tried bargaining with God. Every night I would pray "Please God if you make my grandpa better I will go to church every Sunday, I will give my whole paycheck to the church, or whatever you want. " I actually thought I could bribe God into healing my grandfather. I thought that kind deeds could save my grandfather. What I didn't realize is that God was actually saving my grandfather from the pain of suffering with cancer anymore.

My grandfather's illness was a very long and hard one. He was in and out of the hospital, in and out of hospice, finally on life support. We watched this bigger than life man lose his independence, dignity, and freedom.

As care givers we learned that a point has to come that you have to let go of your loved ones so they can be at peace. You learn to accept gods will. You learn that being angry or bitter or bargaining with god or tears just don't work.

My grandfather in his last days taught us that the ultimate gift of love you can give a person with cancer is the gift of acceptance. Accept that no one lives forever, accept that cancer cannot rob you of the love you have for that person, accept that dying is just another form of living, and accept that your loved one will be ok if you are ok with their diagnosis.

When my grandfather was dying we used to look at family pictures of the time we spent together. As we looked at those pictures I did not realize until after he was gone that each time I remember him I am celebrating his life. I am letting the light of his spirit shine into the world.

Chapter 3

As a caregiver I personally learned that peace only comes for your loved ones and you when you learn to accept what must be. When you waste your time being bitter or angry, or bargaining with god, or fighting over the doctors diagnosis, you are taking away precious time with your loved one.

"A Caregiver's Prayer"

"Lord I pray your angels give me strength when I am weak. A friend to hold me when I feel alone. A peaceful accepting heart when you call my loved one home. Let my loved ones legacy shine in my eyes, let their kind and gentle heart live in my words and actions. Amen."

"It is when God appears to have abandoned us that we must abandon ourselves most wholly to him.' F.Fenelon

When my grandfather died it was almost like my grandmother did also. My grandfather passed away on July 5, 1995. He finally was set free when my grandmother signed the dnr order after weeks of praying for God to lead our family. The day my grandfather died it was a brutally hot and miserable Summer's day. Ironically or maybe mercifully we got to the hospital to see my grandfather late that day. For weeks we had been going to the hospital at a set time to visit grandpa.

 It was on that day that my mom a caregiver herself for the mentally ill had to work overtime at her job.

We had waited for my mom to get out of work so we could all drive to the hospital together.

When we got to the fourth floor of the hospital the door to my grandfather's room was tightly shut.

A young nurse approached us with a very solemn face saying, "I'm sorry Fred passed away a hour ago." Grandma fell apart. Having a heart condition we were afraid she was going to collapse. After calming her down we called the rest of our family to come say goodbye to grandpa. We waited for them to arrive and then went into grandpa's room together.

To our surprise grandpa looked completely and utterly at peace.

As we were planning our grandfathers funeral my mother, grandmother, and I got one more ultimate gift of love from God and my grandfather. We had gone into a flower shop to purchase flowers for the funeral.

My grandmother loved flowers. Her backyard looked like a botanical garden. My grandfather's favorite colors were yellow and red. After we picked out the flowers for the funeral and paid for them we were walking out of the flower shop when the owner called us back. He handed my grandma a yellow rose, and my mom and I red ones. He did not know those were my grandfather's favorite colors!

My grandmother in her very deep pain did not see what we saw in the gift of the flowers until weeks later. My grandfather had a full military funeral on July 7, 1995 and was buried in Calverton national cemetery on Long Island, New York.

After we buried grandpa, grandma felt alone in a crowded room. She could not stop crying, everywhere she looked memories of my grandfather haunted her soul. Grandma became very depressed.

We were very worried about her. After a few months grandma was not getting better. It was not until one day grandma was reading her bible and a scripture turned her tears of mourning into healing rain. The scripture was john 14:1 "Do not let your heart be troubled, trust in God, trust also in me."

Trust, we must trust in our tears. As caregivers our tears are not a sign of weakness or necessary mourning. Our tears can be tears of acceptance, of healing, of peace. It is perfectly acceptable to cry. It is a gift to let our loved ones cry. As caregivers it is important to have an outlet for our feelings or our fears. Seek out others to talk to if you are feeling over whelmed, need advice or just a shoulder to lean on. As much as we want to be superman we are not. We are only human.

We must also remember as caregivers that we must let our loved ones express their feelings. Even though it may be hard for us to hear. Let your loved ones talk about their fears, there wishes, their lives. It is healthy to have a good cry together.

Chapter 4

"Once you chose hope anything possible. "   Christopher reeve.

Hope it's a cancer patient's secret weapon against gloomy lonely days. As my great uncle Willie laid in a hospital dying of lung cancer hope became his best friend. Like my grandfather, my uncle was a strong and proud man. A hard worker who provided for his family. Uncle Willie was a former butcher, at one time in his younger days he drove a team of horses. He was diagnosed with cancer when he was 85 years old. Like my grandfather my uncle was fighting a losing battle with cancer.

As his body weakened his mind did not. Uncle Willie formulated a plan to provide for his family before he passed, to leave us hope after he was gone. As we visited with my dying uncle day after day he reminded us how special we were to him and to god.

He shared with us family history to be passed down to a new generation. As caregivers it is important to be bearers of our family roots, family history and stories. It is important to our loved ones to know that family history will live on. As caregivers we can preserve our family history by making up scrapbooks, recording our loved ones, writing our loved ones thoughts on paper, or making photo albums. It helps our loved ones to know that hope will be passed down. Uncle Willie had a very short battle with cancer, but the lesson we learned from his battle is that everyone needs hope.

Our family's histories contain stories of hope. Hope of seeing our dreams succeed, hope of finding that special someone, hope that our children will grow up happy and healthy.

"You got to live life not think about it. Step into the mist of things. Try and fail and stand and love and learn and forgive, and forget, and be daring, and don't live in fear. " This is the lesson I learned from my bubbly and faithful friend Diana while she was going her battle with liver cancer.

Diana and I met while working together in a collage café. Diana was this incredible loving soul who had a young heart, gave the best advice, and made this to die for chicken salad. Diana was the head cook at the café. When Diana told me she had stage three liver cancer I was at a loss for words. I didn't know what to say, or how to act around Diana. I immediately fell into a caregiver role.

Diana was an independent woman. She was a walker who walked five miles a day, she was much older than me, but I never knew her age. When Diana got sick I started to mother and smother her. I began to crowd her. This independent woman who always took care of herself began to resent how I was treating her. She did not want to be babied.

One day when I was visiting Diana at her apartment, I immediately began to take care of her. I was picking up a pile of her dirty laundry to wash.Diana got mad at me saying, "Why are you treating me like this?"Her words stopped me in my tracks. Turning to Diana I answered honestly, "Because you are sick."

Loving Diana sat me down. "Patti, sometimes the best thing you can do for a person with cancer is nothing at all. Sometimes just being with them is the only thing you can do. "She said.

At that moment Diana's words penetrated my thick skull. People with cancer still want their independence. They don't want their choices taken away from them just because there sick. Sometimes as caregivers we tend to think that we must do everything for a cancer patient, but that just isn't true.

People with cancer want to keep their independence, there freedom, there choices for as long as they can.

As caregivers we must respect their right to choose. Choose their own decisions on health care, final wishes, and other important things. As caregivers we have to sometimes learn to back off and give our loved ones space. Sometimes the best thing we can do is really nothing at all.

Diana's world famous chicken salad recipe.

2 packages of boneless chicken breast

1 large onion chopped chunky

4 stalks of celery finely chopped

2 large tomatoes sliced

4 teaspoons of honey

3 teaspoons of Italian seasoning

1 dill pickle chopped

5 teaspoons of mayonnaise.

Cooked chicken breast in a pot of boiling water for an hour and a half.

Let chicken cool for 20 minutes.

Dice chicken.

In a large mixing bowl add honey, mayonnaise, onion, pickle, Italian seasoning, celery and tomato.

Add chicken.

Mix two more teaspoons of mayonnaise.

Let it chill one hour before serving.

Can be served on rye bread or whole wheat crackers.

Chapter 5

"He placed me in a little cage away from garden's fair but I must sing the sweetest songs because he placed me there. Not beat my wings against the cage it it's my makers will but raise my voice to heaven's gate and sing louder still. " Kyle Sweet.

This was the inspirational poem my dear friend Kyle recited over and over again to help her get through the pain of living with ovarian cancer. Kyle and I never met in person. She was the wife of a Christian rock singer of a band I admired growing up. Kyle was my pen pal. Kyle was the big sister I never had. Our friendship bloomed from being pen pals to spiritual sisters.

Kyle Rae was a very spiritual, giving, kind, and loving person. When I was going through the toughest times in my life Kyle and her husband Michael was there for me. They reached out to me and truly was an example of Christ's love on earth.

Although I was not a direct caregiver to Kyle I learned many lessons from her battle with cancer. Unlike the other people I have known and cared for with cancer Kyle battle was a very public one.

Kyle had to fight cancer every day with cameras and reporters surrounding her. Being a famous makeup artist and wife of a lead singer of a rock band Kyle could have wallowed in self-pity or used her battle to make people feel sorry for her family, but Kyle did not. Kyle my dear friend used her battle to help others fighting cancer.

Kyle talked openly about her struggle. She shared all she was going through. Through the sale of her husband's cds called "Touched." She raised money for cancer research and money for Dana Faber Cancer Institute in Massachusetts.

Kyle became an inspiration not only to her friends but people around the world.

Kyle used music, beautiful poetry, and scripture to touch people's lives and heal the broken hearted.

Kyles spirit, her warmth, her generosity will live on for many years to come. Because I was not living in the same state as Kyle I was not able to be a direct caregiver of her physical needs but I was a caregiver at the same time. How you ask?

We do not have to be with the person physically to be a caregiver. We can be a caregiver for their emotional, spiritual, or financial needs.

For Kyle I became a prayer giver. I prayed for Kyle at a certain time every single day. Sometimes the most powerful gift we can give a person is to simply pray for them.

To simply listen is a gift all by itself. If you have a friend or loved one who is going through this battle and you can't be with them physically there are lots of ways you can help. Another way I supported my friend Kyle was I made the point to send her a card e mail, or letter every week.

For a person battling this disease sometimes all it takes is to get a letter or card to make there'd ay a little brighter. You can also help financially. I am not suggesting you pay medical bills but there are little things that add up to a lot when a family is taking care of a person with cancer.

Below are some suggestions on how to help.

1. Send the family a gift card to a local food store so the family and patient can share a special meal together.

2. If the patient is going for chemo treat the patient to a new bathrobe and slippers. This will make the patient feel like a million bucks.

3. A lot of people don't know that when a person is going through treatment they can't wear perfume, or be around a lot of different smells. Flowers are nice but sometimes it makes the patient sick. So instead of buying flowers but the patient a cd player and one of their favorite cds. This will help ease their soul as they are going through treatment.

4. If the patient is a parent send the children a gift card to a movie and then arrange for a responsible babysitter to take the children to the movies so the patient and there partner can share some quality time together.

5. Offer to pay for a maid service for a week so the caregiver will have one less thing to worry about.

6. If involved in a church group organize some people to do some yard work or cook some meals.

7, Offer to pay for a weeks' worth of gas for the family or patient to get back and forth to the doctor or the hospital.

8. Pay for the parking garage or tolls.

9. Offer to pay for a prescription or one medical supply.

10. Offer to sit with the patient for an hour or two so the caregiver can have some time to decompress.

These are little steps you can take to help a loved one.

The following are a list of places you can donate a love gift to aid in the fight against cancer.

1. Dana Faber Cancer Institute 10 brook line Place west 6th floor brook line, Massachusetts 02445 attn. partners in courage.

2,. Breast Cancer research 60 east 56 th Street 8th floor New York, New York 10022

3. Pediatric Cancer Research 9272 Jerome rd. suite a   -107a Irvine, Calf 92618

4. American Cancer Fund [813] 490 -4700

Chapter 6

"Now the God of hope will fill you with joy and peace in believing that you may abound in hope through the power of the Holy Ghost. "
Romans 15:13

When I met my husband Anthony we were working together at a factory. Just weeks after meeting my new coworker Anthony he left the factory to work at another job. I didn't see Anthony again for 10 years when we met once again on a blind date.

We had our first date at ruby Tuesdays. During our first date we discovered we had many things in common. We became inseparable fell in love quickly, and got engaged just two months after having our first date.The first time I met Anthony's traditional, warm, big Italian family I immediately felt accepted.

Anthony's parents, siblings, aunts, uncles, and cousins became a part of my heart, they became a part of who I am.

Anthony and I got married on Oct. 17, 1999 in a small country church on the east end of Long Island. It was a perfect fall day. The leaves had begun changing colors, there was a crisp chill in the air, but it was not yet winter. Fall embraced us like an old friend.

On that perfect October day I walked down the aisle with both my mom and dad at my side in my long white flowing wedding dress as our churches choir director sang Ava Maria. I saw the faces of my loved ones beaming with love, light, and joy.

Two of those faces were my mom's older sister Roberta and my husband's uncle Al, both of them were loving souls and both were battling cancer.

Aunt Roberta had bone cancer. Uncle Al had kidney cancer. At my wedding both sides of my family were blessed to have made some wonderful memories that day. It was at my wedding that we found out that Anthony's sister Christen was pregnant with her first daughter Kassidy Rose.

It was also at my wedding that both aunt Roberta and uncle Al was able to enjoy this wonderful, magical, carefree time with their family and friends.

As caregivers it is very important for us to realize that the patient needs a large, strong, support system. Families, loved ones, friends, neighbors, church members, and class mates should be allowed to visit the patient for as long as they want, as many times as they want.

As caregivers we must put our personal differences aside with other family members so the patient can enjoy all members of their family.

It is important for us as caregivers to realize that is the patient wants to travel, go to a family event, visit a friend, go to church, that they should not be limited to do so.

As caregivers we tend to want to protect or reserve the patient's energy for fear if they overexert themselves or get upset they may get sicker or break. Not true.

If the patient wants to go and have a picnic, go swimming in the ocean, go to a party, go to a rock concert, let them. It is good for their soul. It is important that they are not reminded 24 hours a day 7 days a week that they have cancer.

We must learn that we can't control the cancer but controlling the patient. Cancer is what it is. The patients should not have to stop living because our fears prevent them from doing so.

Chapter 7

"The bond that links your true family is not of blood but of respect and joy in each other's life." Richard Bach

Everyone has someone in their life that inspires them to greatness. For me personally it is god, my parents, my grandparents, and my fourth grade teacher, Mrs. Esteves.

 Growing up I was a special education student with a learning disability of dyslexia. I was picked on, bullied, and didn't have a lot of self-confidence, until Mrs. Esteves came into my life.

Mrs. Esteves saw in me the gift I had for writing. Mrs. Esteves fueled my passion for writing by encouraging me and helping me overcome my dyslexia. Mrs. Esteves was a true friend. Someone who give the shirt off her back to help someone in need. She was a great teacher.

Long after I became a high school grad Mrs. Esteves and her husband kept in touch with my family and I through letters, e mails and phone calls.

Even after Mr. and Mrs. Esteves retired and moved down to Florida they were still a huge part of my life. The loving couple even attended my wedding.

One spring morning I went to my mail box opened it up and found a letter from Mrs. Esteves inside. Getting one of Mrs. Esteves letters always left me with a warm sunshiny feeling. With the exception of this particular letter. My heart sunk as I read the words, "Mr. Esteves has been diagnosed with blood cancer."

I ran in the house shaking because yet another of my loved ones had been diagnosed.

I broke the tragic news to my husband and parents. We all had a good cry. Tossing and turning in my bed that night I could not sleep. Something that Mrs. Esteves said in that letter ate away at me.

After she broke the news that her beloved husband had cancer she asked me to not write her any more.

I did not understand why. What had I done wrong?

"Good friends are like stars. You don't always see them but always know they are there. "

For weeks I was depressed that Mrs. Esteves was shutting me out at a time she needed her friends the most. I had written her several times after receiving her letter. She did not write back. Her silence tore apart my heart. I prayed for her and Mr. Esteves. I wanted God to give me an answer as to why she didn't want me in her life any more. The answer I was seeking came in a rare and unexpected form.

One of my old class mates had looked me up on line and contacted me. It was a classmate that once had been a big part of my life, but we had nothing in common anymore. As I listened to my classmate ramble on about his boring job I realized that Mrs. Esteves was not trying to hurt me when she wrote what I thought was her final letter to me. We were a beautiful part of each other's past but we were facing two very different futures.

Mrs. Esteves was becoming a full time caregiver trying to squeeze in every last moment she could with her husband. I was traveling down a very different road. My future was full of aspirations and plans.

Mrs. Esteves's future was full of worry, sacrifice, and taking care of a sick husband.

I learned from Mr. Esteve's battle with cancer that sometimes the moving thing you can do is to step out of a person's life and give them the space while they are going through this journey. Sometimes they just need time. Sometimes they just need to be alone to figure out there way through the maze of pain and confusion.

I didn't hear from Mrs. Esteves for two years. And then one day I opened the mail box to find a letter from her.

Mr. Esteves had gone to be with the lord. Mrs. Esteves had found her way back to the person she was before cancer put her life on hold. I know it's not easy to see someone struggling with the beast and to have them shut you out. It may seem like they are being selfish or mean but they are not. They just need time to navigate through the charging waters they are swimming through.

"Jesus healed many who have various diseases." Mark 1:34.

Sometimes the most important lessons in life are the most painful.

In the process of writing this book I met a man, a stranger on the street who touched my heart so deeply that I could not let this moment pass without mentioning him. His name was Peter. Peter was probably in his early thirties. He was in a wheel chair and had survived seven different types of cancer.

From the moment I met Peter I felt his positive energy flowing through him. Peter was a big brother, ran his own company, and bought wheel chairs for people who could not afford them. In front of a Christian book store where I met Peter he taught me a very valuable lesson in forgiveness.

As we chatted Peter revealed to me that when he was diagnosed with cancer his wife could not deal with it and left him for another man. When I asked Peter if he was able to forgive his wife he looked at me and said, "If Jesus was able to forgive my sins, should I not forgive another's?"

As we talked about forgiveness, Peter revealed to me how important it was to him to know he was able to forgive all the people in his life that had hurt him, and how he needed to be forgiven by the people he hurt.

This brings me to a very important conclusion, as caregivers I think we need to make sure the people we are taking care of knows that we have forgiven them for past hurts, mistakes, and grudges.

Forgiveness is very powerful. If you have a terminal illness and feel like you are unforgiving for something you have done it will leave you in turmoil and your heart won't be at peace. If you are dealing with a disease like cancer I believe the best gift you can give your loved ones is to forgive them for hurting you and ask them for forgiveness too.

Chapter 8

Prayer of St. Francis.

"Lord make me an instrument of your peace, where there is hatred let me sow love, where there is injury pardon, where there is doubt, faith, where there is despair hope, where there is darkness light, and where there is sadness joy, father grant that I may not seek to be consoled as to console, to be understood as to understand, to be loved as to love, amen. "

"Humor is our way of defending ourselves from life absurdities by thinking absurdly about them". Lewis Mumford.

"I'm going into the hospital to deliver my twins." my coworker Jane said as she spoke of having her double breast removal. Jane was diagnosed with breast cancer one January day right before coming to work at a day care. Jane, my mom and I all worked together at a day care in Georgia with two year olds.

Jane who always had a smile on her face, a song in her heart, and a spring in her step casually broke the news to us with a positive attitude and humor.

When Jane told us about her cancer it was hard not to believe that Jane would not drag the beast by the hair look it straight in the eye and laugh in its face. Jane would overcome cancer and would use humor to do so. Jane positive attitude kept all of us positive.

She taught us it was ok to laugh at cancer. She taught us that just because a person has cancer it does not mean they have a death sentence. She taught us that god is in control and won't abandon us.

It was Jane that actually held her circle of friends together. She would not let us fall apart. After Jane had her double removal went to visit her at the hospital and she me in stitches. She told me she did not want people to cry for her.

As caregivers and as patients we must remember it is perfectly fine to laugh. Laughter really is the best medicine. I truly believe that it was the laughter of her friends, family, and her own that has made Jane a breast cancer survivor.

Chapter 9

"God heals a poem for breast cancer survivors."

"Remember when you heard the words and you were thrown into a black sea of woe, God heals. Remember in your loneliness and pain, God heals. Remember friends prayers, your families encouragement, glimpses of hope from angels, God heals. Quiet you can hear God whispering now, I will heal. "

Breast cancer resources.

City of Hope Cancer center Los Angeles, California

Phone number 1-800-826-4673

Memorial Sloan Kettering Center New York City

Phone number 1-800-525-2225

Cancer support group

Rabloch Cancer Foundation Inc.

Bloch cancer One H. and R. Block Way

Kansas City, Mo. 64105

Phone number 1-800-433-0464

Locks of Love

234 Southern Blvd.

West Palm Beach, Florida 33405

Phone number 561-833-7332

Cancer care

Phone number 1-800-813-4673

They have offices in New York, New Jersey and Connecticut.

Financial help

1-800-813-Hope

This number offers financial help for people with low income.

Cancer Treatment of America Centers.

Phone number 1-888-767-0247

Counseling

Fran place

Phone number 949-474-4337

Cancer care

Phone number 1-800-813-4673

"When you were born you cried and the world rejoiced. Live your life so that when you die the world cries and you rejoice. " Old Cherokee expression.

Dad, father, Pa, Daddy, all words that make you immediately feel secure, warm, happy, beautiful and loved. My father, my friend, my hero, my confident, my teacher, Bernie Leudeman was a man with no regrets. He loved, he lost, and he lived.

When I think of my father, the Frank Sinatra song," My Way." comes to mind.My father was passionate about life. He was a hard worker, faithful friend, loving father, and devoted husband. He loved gardening just like his mom. He loved animals just like St. Francis. He loved fast cars, cb radios, fish, and music.

Dad wore many hats. He started his working career selling pretzels with his father at Madison Square Garden. Became a proud business owner, and finally retired from Pilgrim State Hospital on Long Island, New York in the early 1990s.

Dad and mom met on a blind date. They got married on August 22,1970 in a beautiful ceremony.

Dad and mom had two children, my brother and I.

Dad was nicknamed "The Bull" because he was a strong strapping man. He had a booming voice, blue eyes and blond hair. He was born on Oct. 25, l942 in Brooklyn, New York and died sept 27, 2006, another victim of cancer.

My dad's death was untimely, shocking, and the most painful for my family. After my parents retired my family moved out of New York to Georgia. Dad always loved cowboys, Westerns, and cowboy music so moving to the Deep South was a dream come true for him.

Chapter 10

"It matters not who you love, where you love, why you love, when you love, or how you love, it only matters that you love." John Lennon.

My parents purchased a charming 3 bedroom 2 bath country ranch with a huge backyard in a lovely small southern town. They quickly became adopted southerners. Dad loved working in his flower garden, playing with his lab in the backyard, and sitting on his porch listening to music. Dad was the picture of perfect health.

In the summer of 2006 my husband and I planned a family reunion. It was my parents 36 wedding anniversary coming up and my younger nieces birthday, they shared the special day.

My in laws, nieces, and my brother flew in from New York for the big event. The family spent the week touring the sights around Atlanta and just having a wonderful time together.

On the day of my parent's anniversary and my nieces birthday we had a fun celebration. We danced, laughed, ate and sang at my house. It was a happy time for all of us.

When the week came to an end we were sad to see the rest of our family go but we knew we would see them again soon. On the way home from dropping our guests off at the airport my dad who was driving started to complain of shoulder pain.

He thought it was arthritis. Dad went home and rested.

The next day my husband and I went to work. When I arrived home there was a message on my answering machine from my mom. "Dad can't move his arm or leg, I think he has had a stroke.", Mom said. My husband and I drove to my parents' home.

We tried to convince my dad to go to the hospital.

Dad refused, just brushing it off.

Later that night my dad got a lot worse. He couldn't walk and was having really bad headaches. We called 911.At the hospital the doctors ran all kinds of tests on dad. I will never forget the moment the doctor came in to my dad's room and told my mom, husband and I that dad had brain cancer and there was nothing they could do. Everything stopped. I remember hearing screams and I didn't even realize the screams were coming from me. I remember my husband almost passing out and my mom turning white as a ghost. Then I remember dad the rock of our family. I remember the exact words he said to the doctor.

"How long do I have?" he asked first.

The young doctor looked at me.My husband wrapped his arms tightly around me. "Maybe a week." The young doctor said. "I want to go home to die', Dad said to mom.

Later that night my brother flew back to Georgia. I remember how devastated he was. We sat in silence as we drove back to my parents' house to wait for hospice to set up a hospital bed for my dad in the living room. I remember my brother and I couldn't look at each other for fear we might burst out in tears. We couldn't comfort each other; there were just no words to say.

The following day my dad came home to the hospice bed. I just fell apart.

Mom, my brother and my husband remained strong.

My dad made clear to us his final wishes. He told us everything he needed to say. There were no words left unspoken between us, no tears unshed, no apologies not given.We had both a Catholic priest and a Methodist priest give dad last rites.

One week to the day my dad was diagnosed with brain cancer, he died.

We were unprepared for this financially, and emotionally. When dad died we had known that he wanted to have a catholic mass because he was a strict catholic and he also wanted my pastor present at the funeral mass. Together the Catholic and Methodist pastors preformed a touching memorial mass to send my dad's soul back to God.

Dad was buried in New York next to his parents.

After dad died I felt lost, betrayed, and very lonely. I was not mentally prepared to lose my dad. I had a really hard time getting over his death.

Talking about my dad helped. Going to places we used to go together helped. Having a picture of him on the dashboard of my car helped.

The most important lesson I learned from my dad's death is that you are never alone in your grief. Even though I felt alone there were people out there to help.

 Everyone goes through the grieving process differently. No one has the right to tell you to stop mourning. I don't care if it has been a day or ten years since you lost your loved one. There is no set amount of time that normal or not normal to grieve for your loved one.

It is the same when you have been diagnosed. Everyone reacts differently to their diagnoses and that is normal. Another lesson I learned from my dad's death is no matter how much pain you are in life will go on. You will find a way to go on.

There are seven stages of grief. They are as follows;

1. Shock

2. Denial

3. Bargaining

4. Guilt

5. Anger

6. Depression

7. Acceptance.

What can you do if you have lost a loved one?

Here are several suggestions to start the healing process.

1. Get plenty of sleep.

2. Exercise.

3. Make sure you eat.

4. Avoid drugs and alcohol.

5. Join a support group.

It is very important at this difficult time that you get sleep. If you wake up feeling exhausted your mind in not capable of helping you heal. You will find yourself more irritable, more depressed, and more sensitive. Sleep helps you relax, and heal the mind.

Exercise. During this time exercise could be the key to healing. It releases stress and tension. It will help you forget your pain.

I know it can be difficult for you to eat right now but your body needs food. Grief expends an enormous amount of energy. Without food your body will become run down and very weak.

Avoid drugs and alcohol. It may help you to forget your pain for a while but the hard cold truth is it won't bring your loved one back. Destroying your own health will only add to your suffering.

Join a support group. There is no shame in admitting your pain. People will understand your pain because they are going through it too.

The following are some examples of how to honor a loved one.

1. Plant a flower garden. For every birthday or anniversary plant a flower in memory of your loved one.

2. Collect funny stories, memories or photos f rom other family members, friends, and colleagues of your loved one and make a special scrapbook honoring what they meant to all of you.

3. Set aside a special place and time to talk to your loved one every day. They are in your heart and always will be.

4. Donate to your loved one favorite charity.

5. Don't stop celebrating your loved ones birthday, anniversary, or special days that meant something to them. Your loved ones are a part of who you are and should be celebrated every day.

As my family, loved ones and I were going through this journey together we found that music really helped us on the days we felt discouraged. The following are a list of songs that I put together to help lift your spirits. These were songs my loved ones used as they were going for treatment, songs we used to give us comfort and peace and to summon our guardian angels.

1. "A Wonderful World" by Louie Armstrong.

2. "Somewhere over the rainbows' by Judy garland.

3. "It's a beautiful day" by U2

4. "It's my life' by Bon Jovi.

5. "True Colors' by Cindy Lauper.

6. "She's got a way' by Billy Joel.

7. "Honestly' by Stryper.

8;" Friends" by Michael W. Smith

9. "I will survive' by Gloria Gaynor.

10. "Peace in the valley' by Elvis.

11. " You are so beautiful' by Joe cocker.

12. "Aint no mountain high enough"by Diana ross.

13. " Walking on sunshine" by Katrina and the Waves.

14. " I'm too sexy" by right said Fred.

15. "Circle of life" by Elton John.

I thought it would be interesting if I added to this book some of my loved ones favorite recipes.

Chocolate dip strawberries.

One bag of semi-sweet chocolate chips.

One pint strawberries, washed.

Place chocolate chips in a medium medal bowl set over a sauce pan of boiling water. Stir until melted. Dip strawberries   let cool. For one hour.

Chicken and Cole slaw wrap.

One can of chunky white chicken meat.

One cup slaw.

One can of crushed pineapple.

Two flour Tostitos.

In a small mixing bowl add chicken, Cole slaw, and pineapple. Stir, cover and refirgete for at least 25 minutes. To serve top each torilla with mixture. Enjoy.

Noodles and barking dogs.

One package of hot dogs.

One box of shells.

One pound of grated American cheese.

Salt and pepper.

Two can s of tomato sauce.

Cook hot dogs in boiling water for ten minutes.

In a separate of boiling water cook shells until soft. Slice hot dogs. In a large tray put one can of tomato sauce on the bottom of the tray. Combine hot dogs cheese, salt and pepper, and shells in a the tray. Put second can of tomato sauce on top. Bake at 400 degrees for 45 minutes.

Throughout my loved ones battle with the beast we prayed a lot. The following are scriptures that gave us the most strength, encouragement and comfort while we were in our valley.

Chapter 11

"Which is Christ in you the hope of glory."

Colossians 1:27

"He shall deliver the in six troubles, yea in seven there shall know evil touch thee." Job 5: 19

"My flesh and my heart may fail but god is the strength of my heart and my portion forever". Psalm 73:26

"For the Lord said unto the house of Israel seek yea me and ye shall live." Amos 5:4

"For by the grace are ye saved through faith and not of yourself it is God's gift." Ephesians 2: 8

"Be of good courage and he shall strengthen your heart all that hope in the Lord." Psalm 31:24

"Though shall make thy prayer unto him and he shall hear thee." Job 22:27

"I will see you again and your heart shall rejoice and your joy no man will steal." John 16:22

"For you will light my candle, the Lord God will enlighten my darkness." Psalm 18:28

'Yet if any man suffer as a Christian let him not be ashamed but let him glorify God on his behalf." Peter 4:16

"For I will restore health unto you and I will heal you of thy wounds said the Lord.' Jeremiah 30:17

"Fear not." Kings 6:16

Before I close this book I have one more thing I would like to discuss. That is how to thank a caregiver. Here is a list of suggestions on how to thank the doctors, nurses, home health aides, pastors, and therapists.

1. Mention care givers name in a Thanksgiving blessing.

2, Give the caregiver a day off with pay.

3, Send the caregiver a little gift and include in a note why they are such a special caregiver.

4. Send food to the facility where the caregiver works.

5. Make a donation in the caregivers name.

6, Simply say thank you.

"Cancer Can't"

Cancer cant cripple love.

It can't shatter hope.

It can't corrode faith.

It can't eat away hope.

It can't destroy confidence.

It cannot kill friendship.

It cannot fade memories.

It cannot invade the soul.

It cannot reduce eternal life.

It cannot quench your inner light.

It cannot steal your spirit.

It cannot lesson the power of gods healing.

Cancer can make you stronger.

It can make you treasure every sunset.

It can make you pray.

It can make you believe in miracles.

It can make you see yourself through god's eyes.

My daily diary. Use this to write down scripture, prayers, feelings, or thoughts.

1. I am beautiful because .

2. I can beat cancer because.

3. My battle with cancer will help others because.

4. Scriptures that encourage me are.

5. My cancer battle song is.

6. The reasons I will not give up are.

7. I have hope because.

8. My prayer is.

9. Lessons I learned from cancer are.

10. A message I want to tell my family.

11. My final wishes are.

12. My favorite songs are.

13. What I want the world to know about me is .

14. Things that give me peace are.